The Ketogenic Diet

Beginner's Guide to Rapid Weight Loss and Unlimited Energy

The information herein is offered for informational purposes solely, and is universal as so. The presentation of the information is without contract or any type of guarantee assurance.

The trademarks that are used are without any consent, and the publication of the trademark is without permission or backing by the trademark owner. All trademarks and brands within this book are for clarifying purposes only and are the owned by the owners themselves, not affiliated with this document.

Table of Contents

Introduction

I want to thank you and congratulate you for downloading this book, *The Ketogenic Diet: Beginner's Guide to Rapid Weight Loss and Unlimited Energy.*

This book contains proven steps and strategies on how to lose weight and gain energy in a very short period of time. It also teaches you how to sustain this new lifestyle. The results will astound you. You will feel better than you have in years. You will gain mental clarity. As your body rids itself of harmful sugars, it will transform into a fat burning machine. Enjoy this process and be proud of yourself for taking this step towards optimum health and well-being.

Chapter One:
Welcome to the Wonderful World of Ketones!

Weight and diet. For the majority of us, these words evoke shame and frustration. We are not alone: eight out of ten men and women over the age of 18 are either bothered by their weight or are actively on a diet. Unfortunately, there is no specific recipe for success, and many people are lured in by fad diets which can cost a high amount of money and produce minimal results. The key to weight loss is a diet which is based upon physiology and science, not supplements and false claims. A ketogenic diet targets the root cause of the weight gain: hormones. Imbalanced insulin and high blood sugar levels result in extreme hunger and drastically low energy levels, putting dieters at a disadvantage right from the start. A ketogenic diet immediately focuses on lowering sugar levels in our body which helps you feel healthier and more energized almost immediately.

A Little Biology

After we consume sugar and starch (carbohydrates) these foods are broken down into sugar (insulin and glucose) in our blood. If these levels become too high, our bodies start to store fat in the blood cells, which results in weight gain. But when glucose levels are low, the body starts to burn fat and produces ketones. As ketones levels rise, blood cells start eating away at fat, and you enter a state of ketosis. This means you are burning more fat than you are consuming, which results in quick and consistent weight loss. The goal of the ketogenic diet is to keep you in this metabolic state, and this is achieved by following a low-carbohydrate, high-fat diet.

What is the Ketogenic Diet?

Many nutritional research studies report that following a ketogenic diet results in rapid weight loss and offers many other health benefits. You do not have to count calories on this diet nor do you have to starve yourself. A ketogenic diet, also known as a keto diet, includes foods which are high in natural fats and moderate protein but severely restricts the number of carbs you eat each day. This dietary change eats away at fat in the body while giving you a consistent high level of energy, which also results in weight loss.

The average person's intake of harmful carbohydrates (white bread, pasta, white rice, sugar-sweetened beverages, etc.) ranges between 40-60% of their daily diet. We know this results in obesity; and it also causes a large range of other physical ailments. On a keto diet, carbs only provide 5% of daily food consumption; while protein and healthy fats are 20% and 75%, respectively.

Ketogenic Diet vs. Low-Fat/Low-Calorie Diet

Until recently, we were always told the best way to lose weight, in addition to exercise, was to restrict our caloric and fat intake. For decades, people were eating "diet food" which consisted of highly processed, non-organic ingredients; void of taste and nutritional value. Eating this kind of food leads to metabolic diseases, produces minimal results and is extremely hard to stick with consistently. After decades of this ineffective nutritional plan, doctors and nutritionists started to realize that not all calories are the same. Calories from carbohydrates damage the body, while calories from protein actually help alleviate many physical ailments. Gone are the days of fat-free and low-calorie diets, which are laden with carbohydrates and unpronounceable ingredients. Study after study have found that people on a ketogenic diets lose more than double the number of pounds compared to people on a low-calorie/low-fat diet. Also, keto dieters are more likely to incorporate the diet into their lifestyle than those restricting calories and fat.

Other Health Benefits

There are numerous health benefits to a following a keto diet. Many nutritional studies report that not only is this diet extremely effective for weight loss, it can also drastically improve other health conditions.

- Heart disease

- Diabetes

- Blood pressure

- Acid reflux

- Cancer and tumor growth

- Epilepsy

- Parkinson's disease

- Alzheimer's disease

- Neurological conditions

- Acne

Before starting the ketogenic diet, please check with your physician, especially if you have kidney or heart problems.

As with any diet, the adaptation process can be a challenging one. Fortunately, with the ketogenic diet, your hard work will produce quick results, and you will feel better and more energized than you ever have.

Chapter Two:
Preparing Yourself

The health benefits of following a high-fat, moderate protein and low-carb diet are significant and could ultimately be life-saving. Keep in mind that implementing the ketogenic diet into your lifestyle may be a challenging one. Reading this book indicates that your overall health is important to you, and with hard work come great rewards. Always give yourself credit for taking the steps necessary to reach your goals, even if they feel like small steps to you. Every personal victory, big or small, should be celebrated. And because you made the right decision to follow a ketogenic diet, you will be astounded at how quickly you lose weight, and your goals will be accomplished long before imagined.

Basic Ketogenic Rules

Here are the basic keys to success to give you an overall feel for what a ketogenic diet entails.

Food ratio: 60-75% of your daily food consumption should come from fat, 15-30% from protein and 5-10% of your calories from carbohydrates. For optimal results, try to eat between 20-30 grams of carbs a day, though you may start at 50 grams and work your way down over a week.

Protein intake: You shouldn't be eating more protein than healthy fats. Unlike other low-carb diets, the keto diet does not have you protein-load. Be conscious of this, otherwise you will find it extremely difficult to reach ketosis and lose weight.

Healthy fats: This is where the bulk of your calories come from. Healthy fats include: saturated fats, monosaturated fats and omega 3 fatty acids. A list of the best healthy fats for you to incorporate into your diet is in chapter four.

No need to count calories: A ketogenic diet demands that you be mindful of what your body is telling you. If you are hungry, eat. If you feel full, push the plate away. The right combination of fat, protein and carbohydrates acts like a natural appetite suppressant, which means you eat less at each meal.

Drink water: Remember to drink water consistently throughout the whole day. This is extremely important to aid in hunger suppression and help the body rid itself of toxins. You should aim to drink 10-12 8 oz. glasses a day.

Preparations

There are a few things you should take care of before starting a ketogenic diet. Adequate preparation will help you make this transition smoothly, and every step in this process is imperative for success.

Determine your ideal body weight: On the ketogenic diet, you can set your own target weight, depending upon what feels comfortable to you. If you are unsure what your ideal body weight should be, you can find many calculators online which will tell you what weight is healthiest for you. A very helpful one is: *www.rush.edu/health-wellness/quick-guides/what-is-a-healthy-weight.*

Calculate your daily caloric intake: Now that you have determined how many pounds you want to lose; the next step is to establish the number of calories you cannot eat more than a day. The following online link is the best resource to help you determine how much you should be eating: www.cimedicalcenter.com/metabolism-p124

Calculate amount of protein, carbs and fat needed each day:
This part involves math and may seem confusing at first. But once you understand the reasoning and start calculating, it will make more sense. Important: To convert pounds to kilograms, divide your ideal weight by 2.2. Protein and carbohydrates have 4 calories per gram, and fats have 9 calories per gram.

- Protein: Protein intake should be between 1 and 1.5 grams per kilogram of your ideal body weight. Follow this example:

  A person has a target weight of 100 pounds (we are using this number because it makes calculations easier to understand). First we need to convert pounds to kilograms.

  100 lbs./2.2= 45 kilograms

  45 x 1= 45 grams of protein

  45 x 1.5= 67.5 grams of protein

  The optimal protein intake for this person then would be between 45-68 grams per day. Since protein has 4 calories per gram, this equals 180-272 calories a day from protein.

- Carbohydrates: Men should generally stay under 60 grams a day, women 40 grams. If you are not losing weight, limit your carb intake to 30 grams or less.

- Fats: Fats will make up the majority of your daily calories. This can be calculated easily after you know how much protein and carbs to eat.

- Let's put it all together:

  A person has a target weight of 150 pounds and needs to consume 1800 calories a day.

  -Protein: 150 lbs./2.2=68 kilograms

  68 x 1=68 grams of protein

  68 x 4= 272 calories

  -Carbs: 30 grams x 4= 120 calories

  Add protein calories and carb calories= 392 calories

  -Fat: 1800 total calories- 392 calories= 1408 fat calories

  To convert calories to grams, divide by 9

  1408/9= 156 grams of fat a day

The good news is there is a much easier way to figure this all out (also taking into account your daily activity level). KetoDiet Buddy will do the math for you. Visit: http://ketodietapp.com/Blog/page/KetoDiet-Buddy. But it still good to know the math so you are the most informed about the transformation your body is about to make.

Buy a journal: You must track what you eat after each meal or snack. Start with the number of calories you are allotted each day, and subtract the calories each time you eat. This way you can plan your meals as the day goes on, to ensure you aren't overeating or undereating (undereating on a ketogenic diet will not result in weight loss). You also want to record how you feel throughout the day, as physical mindfulness is very important part of this process. And if you "cheat" or completely fall off the wagon and are unsure as to why, try journaling your feelings and corresponding actions; this may help identify what may have triggered you. Keep recipes you particularly enjoyed in your journal, for easy reference.

Stay accountable: Tell a friend or family member what you are doing. Explain the basics of a ketogenic diet, so they understand the process. Talk about your goals and your fears to help you stay motivated and supported. If there is a social event where food will be served, let this person know of your plans in case you want to call them. This can be extremely helpful if you are having a weak moment. Distraction will help keep your mind off the cravings. Look at this person as your keto sponsor.

Be proactive: Most of our social interactions are focused around food and meals. We go out to lunch with our friends, have beers with our buddies, are tempted by cake at birthday parties, etc. And don't forget the holidays. Have strategies in your back pocket (including one above) so you stay on track. The first few weeks are going to be the most difficult as your body is transforming into a fat-burning machine. It is advised not start this diet right before the holiday season or before a major event.

Kitchen do-over: This part may seem extreme, but you do not want to set yourself up for failure before you even start. Go through the fridge, pantry, cupboards or anywhere else you keep food (time to get the candy stash from under your bed!) and get rid of all high-carb foods. Donate unopened items to your local food pantry or give them to your carb-consuming friends. If there are people in your household who are not following a ketogenic diet, talk to them about the importance of your dietary change and try to keep your food separate from theirs. The following is a list of foods which are advised not to eat while following a ketogenic diet:

- Anything which contains sugar, including:

    -White, brown, cane, raw and confectioner's sugar

    -Syrups, including: maple, carob, corn, caramel and fruit

    -Honey and agave

    -Fructose, glucose, maltose, dextrose and lactose

- All grain products, including:

    -Bread products (sliced bread, bagels, rolls, muffins, etc.)

    -Pasta

    -Crackers, chips, pretzels and candy

    -Cookies, cakes, pies and ice cream

    -Pancakes, waffles

    -Oatmeal and cereals

    -Granola bars

    -Rice products (white, brown, jasmine, quinoa, couscous, pilaf, etc.)

- All corn products, including:

  -Popcorn

  -Tortillas

  -Grits, polenta and corn meal

- Starchy vegetables, including:

  -Corn

  -Peas

  -Potatoes (white, red, sweet, etc.)

  -Artichokes

  -Okra

  -Carrots and parsnips

- Beans (chick peas, kidney, lima, black, brown, lentils, etc.)

- All fruit (fresh, frozen or dried)

- Canned soups, boxed foods, any pre-packaged meal

- Caloric beverages, including:

  -Alcohol (beer, wine, liquor, etc.)

  -Milk (soy, almond, coconut, lactaid, cream, half and half, etc.)

  -Fruit juices

-Soda (though diet soda in moderation is allowed)

- Any foods labeled "low-fat," of "fat-free"

- And foods labeled "low-carb" (because these commercially produced products include preservatives and artificial ingredients)

- Condiments (ketchup, salsa, sour cream, mustard, hot sauces, Worcestershire sauce, etc.)

At this point, you probably feel like there is nothing left to eat. This is far from the truth; you are just changing what you eat. In the next chapter, you will learn what foods and beverages to re-stock your fridge and pantry with. It is going to feel liberating to throw away bad foods and replace them with items of ultimate nutrition. Also, keep in mind, this doesn't mean you will never get to eat the foods listed above again. Once you reach your target weight, you can start incorporating carbs back into your diet. So, you don't have to say goodbye forever; this is just a temporary break.

Reading Nutritional Labels

There is a wealth of information on nutrition labels, but you do not need to decipher it all to fully understand what you are eating. Here is what to focus on when reading a nutritional label:

Serving Size: This information is probably the most important on the label. If a package says it has 4 servings per container, then make sure you are only eating ¼ of what is in the package at a time in order to get amount of fat, protein, and carbohydrates as shown on the label.

Total Calories: Though you won't be counting calories while on the ketogenic diet, it is still a good idea to be acquainted with general numbers.

Total Fat: You should pay attention to the amount of trans fats on the label. Saturated fat is the "good" fat, while trans fats should be consumed in smaller amounts, regardless of if you are dieting or not.

Total Carbohydrates: Look at the total amount first. It if seems high to you, trust your gut and put the item away. Next, dietary fiber is a "good" carb, because it does not raise glucose levels in the body. So you do not have to count dietary fiber when counting carbohydrate grams. Subtract the amount of dietary fiber from the total number of carbs, and this will be the amount of "bad" carbs in the package of food. This is the number you want to pay attention to.

Total Protein: Aim to achieve the daily protein intake as calculated previously, but if you workout aim to slightly increase your protein intake.

Take a deep breath. This chapter was filled with a lot of information, and it is normal to feel overwhelmed. Take it step by step and at your own pace. The better prepared you are, the easier this transition will be. Take pride because you are choosing to improve your physical health and keep reading so you can start losing weight immediately!

Chapter Three:
Keto Diet Side Effects

This chapter is not meant to deter or worry you. While ketogenic diets are safe and have many health benefits, you may experience some negative symptoms at the beginning. This is normal; your body is adjusting to a major dietary change and needs time to adapt. Remember, these side effects will not last forever, and soon they will be replaced by energy and satisfaction as the pounds start falling off.

The Keto Flu

There is no specific "flu" you may catch while on a ketogenic diet. You will not have a cough or a fever. But once you start eating differently, your body will start reacting to this major change. If you are overweight, then your body is used burning glucose. Now you will be training your body to burn ketones instead, and it needs time to adapt. More people than not will feel these flu-like symptoms during the first week after starting the keto diet. These symptoms include:

- Headache

- Fatigue/lack of energy

- Poor sleep

- Nausea

- Feeling brain fogginess

- Upset stomach

Try not to get discouraged. The keto flu is not a pleasant experience, but it is normal and part of the transition to a healthy, slimmer you. Here is a list of remedies which will help feel better:

Drink plenty of H2O: It is very easy to become dehydrated while on a ketogenic diet. Always keep a bottle of water with you to sip on throughout the day. Do not chug water all at one time just to reach your daily intake. This is ineffective, because your body cannot absorb large amounts of water in such a short period of time, and you might flush out important minerals through your urine.

Eat more fat: Remember, the basis of the ketogenic diet is low carbs and high fat. Since carbohydrates will not be your main energy source anymore, you must make sure you are eating enough fat to avoid feeling tired and fatigued. Here are the foods with the lowest carbs and highest fat:

- Fatty red meat

- Bacon

- Cheese

- Chicken with skin

- Cream

- Butter

- Egg yolks

- Nuts, especially macadamia

Eat less protein: The body can change protein to glucose which means if you eat too much of it while in the beginning stage of the keto diet, it will slow down your body's transition into ketosis. Eat more fatty meat, cheese and condiments such a mayonnaise.

Avoid sugar-free foods: As mentioned before, you should try to avoid as many processed and artificial ingredients as possible when making food choices. Since your body is trying to break its dependence on carbs and sugars, it might make sense to buy foods that claim they are sugar or calorie free. Do not do this! It will confuse your system and keep your body craving sugar.

Get moving: When someone is suffering from the flu, usually the last thing they want to do is exercise, or even get out of bed. Your energy levels will be lower than usual during this stage, so don't do anything too strenuous. But you want to keep your body moving, or your body will start conserving fat to retain energy. You want your body to be doing the opposite of this!

Replenish your electrolytes: As mentioned above, drinking a large amount of water each day is important while on a ketogenic diet. Unfortunately, when we drink a lot of water, we are flushing essential electrolytes out of our system at a high speed. This may lead to a magnesium, potassium or sodium deficiency. Here are symptoms of each and how to replenish them:

- Magnesium deficiency symptoms: muscle cramps, dizziness, fatigue

- Foods high in magnesium: nuts, fish, spinach, artichokes

- Potassium deficiency symptoms: depression, heart irregularity, high blood pressure, muscle weakness, constipation

- Foods high in potassium: nuts, avocados, mushrooms, salmon

- Sodium deficiency symptoms: headache, nausea, vomiting, muscle spasms, seizures

- Foods high in sodium: beef broth, bacon, added table salt to meals

Supplement your diet: In addition to electrolytes, there are other dietary supplements you should consider taking to alleviate negative symptoms:

- B and C vitamins (take in large quantities: 1000-2000% of RDA): This will help alleviate tiredness and fatigue.

- Co-enzyme Q10 with L-Carnitine: This has been proven to speed up your body's transition into ketosis.

- Chromium: Blood sugar levels stabilizer and chromium may reduce cravings.

Bad Breath

You may not care that much about this side effect, but the people around you might! The bad breath associated with the ketogenic diet is caused by a specific ketone called acetone, which is produced by the liver when fat starts to metabolize. Once your body is in ketosis, it needs less acetone than usual, so your body naturally gets rid of it through your breath. You may find your urine and sweat smelling of acetone also. Acetone does not have the most pleasant smell (think about nail polish remover) but don't worry, it should go away within a couple weeks.

Digestive Issues

People usually experience some level of GI distress when they make any changes to their diet. On a ketogenic diet, most people report they become constipated and experience low to moderate stomach cramping. You could also get diarrhea, though this is not as common. Up your water intake and make sure you are still following the diet. Your body will regulate itself over time.

Elevated Heart Rate

Some keto dieters experience heart palpitations, comparable to feeling anxious. This should only happen for the first week of the diet, and can also be attributed to dehydration, low sodium level or drinking too much coffee. If this continues for more than a few weeks it is advised you talk to your physician, because this could indicate a pre-existing or dangerous condition.

Rare but Serious Side Effects

The following side effects are very uncommon, though being on a ketogenic diet increases your risk of:

- Ketoacidosis: This occurs in people with diabetes and happens when blood sugar is too high for too long. One case was reported by a woman who was breast feeding at the time.

- Kidney stones: A small number of children developed kidney stones while following a ketogenic diet to help with epilepsy.

- Heightened cholesterol levels: Some people may experience increased LDL and total cholesterol levels.

The benefits of a ketogenic diet are abundant. In a short period of time, you will completely transform your body, improve your health and feel better overall. While being in ketosis is safe, remember all the changes your body is going through. Pay close attention to your body and understand the root cause of any negative symptoms. These effects are temporary and should go away within a week or two. If you feel a higher level of physical distress, contact your doctor. You know your body better than anyone else, and the utmost precautions need to be taken.

Chapter Four:
Let's Shop!

This when you get to restock your fridge and pantry! Hooray! You are going to refer back to this chapter often throughout your journey, especially in the beginning stages. Here we will discuss what rules you have to follow on a daily basis in order to achieve optimal health and promote fast weight loss. Remember not to go over your carbohydrate, protein and fat limit, which you calculated in chapter two.

Rule One: When you feel hungry, eat

Here is a list of protein sources for you to choose from. Eat slowly, and when you feel full, stop eating.

- Meat: beef, pork, bison, goat, wild game, veal. Grass fed meat is preferable, because it is higher in quality omega 3 fats.

- Poultry: turkey, chicken, quail, pheasant, hen, goose, duck.

- Fish: tuna, trout, anchovies, bass, shrimp, scallops, flounder, mackerel, salmon, sardines, mahi-mahi, calamari, snapper

- Shellfish of any kind: clams, shrimp, mussels, scallops, squid, oysters, crab

(Stay away from imitation crab meat, because it contains high amounts of additives)

- Eggs in any way: deviled, fried, hard-boiled, poached, omelets, scrambled, soft-boiled.

- Bacon and sausage

- Soy products: tofu, edamame, tempeh. These foods may be high in carbohydrates, so read labels carefully.

- Canned foods: tuna, salmon. Make sure no extra sugars have been added.

You can prepare the food listed above in a way which suits you. Cook in a variety of ways: bake, sauté, grill, roast, boil, stir-fry; you can even fry your food as long as you coat your food in a keto-approved way, as shown below under Fats to use for cooking.

Rule Two: Eat your veggies!

You must eat 1-2 cups of the following foods each day. Rule of thumb: 1 cup is the same size as a closed fist, and 3 oz. of protein is the size of a deck of cards.

- Cabbage

- Chives

- Greens: beet, collards, mustard, turnip

- Lettuce: arugula, Boston, chicory, endive, escarole, fennel, radicchio, romaine, sorrel

- Parsley

- Spinach

- Kale

- Chard

- Leeks

Consume 1 cup of fibrous vegetables each day. You can choose from more than one item on the list, but make sure the total amount does not exceed 1 cup. The asterisk indicates a food which is higher in sugar and should be limited to ½ cup.

- Asparagus

- Bamboo shoots

- Bean sprouts

- Bell pepper

- Bok choy

- Broccoli

- Brussel sprouts

- Cauliflower

- Carrots*

- Celery

- Cucumber

- Green beans

- Jicama

- Mushrooms

- Okra

- Radishes

- Rhubarb

- Snow peas

- Sugar snap peas*

- Summer squash

- Tomatoes*

- Turnip

- Wax beans

- Water chestnuts

- Zucchini

Rule Three: Good fats are your friends

The following list are recommended fats for you to use. Remember, this is the largest portion of your diet so having a large variety will keep you satisfied and your palate happy.

Fats to use for cooking:

- Butter

- Chicken fat

- Duck fat

- Ghee

- Extra virgin olive oil, cold pressed

- Coconut butter, coconut oil, coconut cream from concentrate

- Red palm oil, limited amounts

Fats to use for cold dressings:

- Avocado oil

- Macadamia oil

- Mayonnaise (make sure it does not contain sugar, or make your own)

- Seed and nut oils: almond, sesame, flaxseed

- Avoid vegetable oils, or use very minimally: grapeseed, sunflower, corn, rice, canola, safflower

Other fats:

- Peanut butter, unsweetened and natural

- Almond butter, unsweetened and natural

- Dark chocolate, 85% or higher cacao content

Rule Four: Foods to eat in limited quantities

The following foods are allowed on a ketogenic diet, but should not exceed the quantities listed.

Cheese: You can eat up to 4 oz., and the carb amount should be less than 1 g/serving.

- Hard cheese: swiss, cheddar

- Soft cheese: brie, camembert, goat, blue, mozzarella, cottage, mascarpone

- Cream cheese: block and whipped

- Processed cheeses are prohibited

Dairy cream: You can eat up to 4T/day, as long as there is no whey in the ingredients.

- Heavy cream

- Whipping cream

- Sour cream

- Full-fat milk

- Avoid half-n-half, because it has too many carbs

Fatty vegetables:

- Olives: up to 7 a day

- Avocado: ½ per day

Mayonnaise: You can eat up to 4 tablespoons a day, but as mentioned above make sure there is no added sugar (less than 1g carbohydrates/serving)

Nuts: Nuts and seeds are a great source of protein and healthy fats, but should only be eaten in small amounts because they are also high in calories and carbs per serving. Here are the nuts with the lowest net carbs:

- Macadamias

- Pecans

- Almonds

- Walnuts

Here are the nuts which are higher in carbs, so eat with caution:

- Cashews

- Pistachios

- Chestnuts

Other condiments:

- Lemon/lime juice: no more than 4t/day

- Ketchup: reduced sugar, 1 T/day

- Soy sauce: up to 4 tablespoons a day

- Salad dressing: Avoid already made salad dressing. It is easy to mix together vinegar, oil and spices to your taste. To make a creamier dressing, use sour cream in place of the vinegar and oil (thin out with a littler water)

- Pickles: no more than 2 servings/day

- Spices: average amount

- Stevia: average amount

Baking: Avoid anything made from whey protein. Small amounts of nut flours is fine, but be careful it isn't listed high on the ingredients list.

Rule Five: Keep hydrated with these choices

- Almond milk, unsweetened: no more than 2 cups/day

- Soy milk, unsweetened: no more than 2 cups a day

- Coconut milk, unsweetened: no more than 2 cups/day

- Bouillon or light broth (this is helpful with electrolyte maintenance)

- Decaf coffee, unsweetened (caffeine can raise blood sugar levels)

- Decaf or herbal tea, unsweetened

- Water

- Lemon and lime juice in small amounts

- Seltzer water, flavored, unsweetened

Rule Six: Stay sweet with these sweeteners

Once your body becomes used to a low-carb diet, your sugar cravings will diminish over the first week. But, if you can't seem to shake the cravings, you can use the artificial sweeteners listed here:

- Splenda, liquid (the powdered has maltodextrin in it)

- Stevia liquid (the powder has maltodextrin in it)

- Xylitol

- Erythritol

Many fruits also supply natural sweetener to your palate. Generally, fruits are too high in carbohydrates to be eaten on a ketogenic diet. But the fruit listed below can be used in small amounts to help with possible sugar cravings.

- Raspberries

- Blueberries

- Strawberries

- Watermelon

Chapter Five:
Meal and Snack Ideas

Now that you are almost a ketogenic diet pro, it is time to put all of this knowledge together and start eating. This chapter will provide you with a sample keto meal plan for one week and several snack ideas.

Go-to snacks

- Salami, turkey or ham, along with a slice of cheese, with mayo or cream cheese spread, rolled up

- Cook bacon and add diced tomato, mayo or cream cheese and roll in a leaf of lettuce

- Cook steak, chicken or pork into bite-sized pieces and mix with mayo, cream cheese, sour cream or a smashed avocado

- Hard boil eggs, mix cooked yolk with mayo or cream cheese

- Smoked salmon with scrambled eggs, topped with dill

- Shrimp mixed with chopped onion, mayo, and dill with sliced cucumbers to dip with

- Jerky (beef or turkey)

- Antipasto with olives, salami, peppers, prosciutto, cheese

- Cook tuna, shred, mix with mayo, eat with pepper slices

- Feta cheese stuffed olives

- Roasted or raw nuts

- Pickles with cheese

- Pork rinds (really!), either on their own or dip in a chopped tomato and sour cream mixture

- Turnip, jicama or radishes sticks dipped in sour cream and spice dressing

- Bake chicken wings with butter, serve with a mixture of blue cheese and sour cream

- Stuff celery with cream cheese and curry spice

- Celery filled with peanut butter or almond butter

- Fry nuts in butter and sprinkle with cinnamon

- Roast pecans, serve with blue cheese and sour cream mixture

- Chunks of avocado mixed with mayo and diced tomatoes

- Steam shrimp, dice, mix with mayo and spices

- Pepperoni slices and cheddar cheese

- Shrimp mixed sour cream and hot chili sauce, sprinkle with cilantro

- Mix ¼c cup of a nut butter with cream cheese

Sample Ketogenic Meal Plan

Monday

- Breakfast: Eggs with tomatoes and sliced bacon

- Lunch: Diced chicken with salad greens, cheese and olive oil

- Dinner: Scrod, cooked in butter, with broccoli

Tuesday

- Breakfast: Eggs with goat cheese, diced tomatoes and fresh basil

- Lunch: Peanut butter mixed with whole milk and stevia milkshake

- Dinner: Beef meatballs, cottage cheese and asparagus

Wednesday

- Breakfast: A ketogenic milkshake (see below)

- Lunch: Greens tossed with diced shrimp, avocado and olive oil

- Dinner: Pork chops fried with butter, spinach with vinegar

Thursday

- Breakfast: Scrambled eggs with chopped onion, tomatoes, avocado and cilantro

- Lunch: Almonds mixed with mashed avocado and chopped tomatoes

- Dinner: Ham steak topped with cheddar cheese and cauliflower

Friday

- Breakfast: Celery stuffed with peanut butter, cottage cheese

- Lunch: Stir-fried chicken cooked in oil and butter with vegetables of choice

- Dinner: Egg fried in butter with bacon and cheese

Saturday

- Breakfast: Ham topped with a fried egg

- Lunch: Sliced almonds and cheese rolled into turkey slices

- Dinner: Shrimp cooked with egg and spinach

Sunday

- Breakfast: Omelet with pepperoni and mushrooms

- Lunch: Roast beef slices with cheese and avocado

- Dinner: Turkey with smashed berries and stevia

Ketogenic Peanut Butter Milkshake

Ingredients

2 tablespoon peanut or any other nut butter

½ cup milk (almond, soy, whole, heavy cream, etc.)

1 tablespoon pure vanilla extract

1 cup ice

Stevia to taste

Put all ingredients in a blender and blend until smooth.

The ideas in this chapter are the building blocks and solutions to generate rapid weight loss and unleash unlimited energy. Some of the snack combinations may seem strange and unappetizing, but keep an open mind. You never know what your taste buds may be craving and some combinations will pleasantly surprise you. There is a wealth of ketogenic and low-carb recipe books available, so do lots of experimenting and don't be afraid to be daring. Food will stop being your nemesis and become the fuel to turn your body into a fat burning machine. Be sure to check out keto diet blogs and public forums to become a part of the ketogenic community, where you can share recipes, tips and tricks, and gain support. It is also very motivating to see success stories to help you gain and maintain confidence. And sooner than later, you will be proudly sharing your own successes for the world to see.

Conclusion

Thank you again for downloading this book!

I hope this book got you excited to start the ketogenic diet. Now you have the information and tools needed to succeed. Remember to take things slowly and if something is confusing to you at first, that's okay. The keto diet takes understanding, patience and dedication. But you will be surprised with how quickly you adapt to this new lifestyle and start shedding the pounds.

The next step is to get off your butt, go shopping and get eating! You can do this!

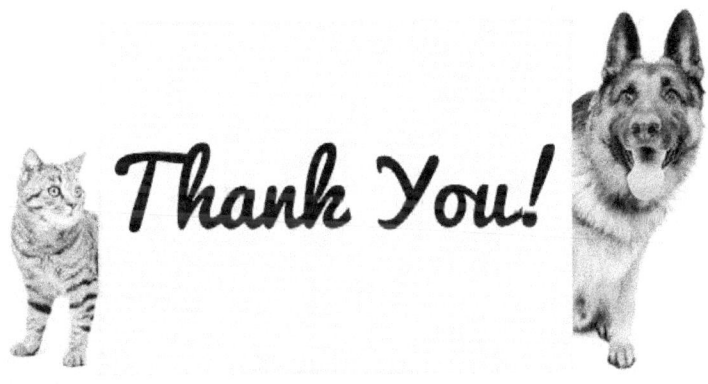

Finally, if you enjoyed this book, then I'd like to ask you for a favor, would you be kind enough to leave a review for this book on Amazon? It'd be greatly appreciated!

Thank you and good luck!